I0440642

Health Food Cures

Kimmy Nelson

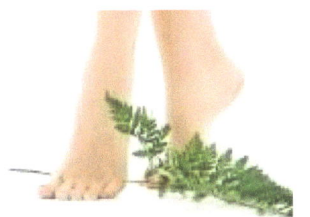

In Dedication to my wonderful

parents Marty and Bill Gerred~

Two of the greatest souls ever!

"I've Known Kim Gerred now for several years and I highly recommend all the works of Kim Gerred and furthermore she is very intelligent & learned so please purchase her books online as soon as possible. You will be so much more informed and educated on this topic."

Dr. Hans J. Petermann PHD 2nd Physics Institute Vienna, Austria MA Degree in German Physical Sciences. Professor, Author & Inventor of the Magnetic Generator & Motor www.MullerPower.com

Because this is a personal home health care guide we have left some blank pages for you to journal personal notes on or on each page for you to write in your own preferences or other tips that help you or your family members.

Use it like a living health journal of recipes and remedies for your family's home health care.

This book is a result of some medical conditions that were not treatable by traditional prescription medicine or the side effects of prescription medicine worsened the conditions of the ailments.

And in one case Prescription medicine caused the illness and that particular prescription has been removed from the market now for being known to cause heart disease, strokes and heart attacks.

Some of the remedies were prescribed by medical doctors who treat pain and some recommendations were from specialists like my primary care physician who treated me at the time of my hospital stay in 2001 who is a licensed M.D.D.O.

And other type of medical doctors such as herbalists, traditionalists, homeopathic doctors (like me) and even an Ortho Molecular doctor also has a part in some of the nutritional remedies that are given in this print. In this edition of "Health Food Cures" we recommend that you drink lots of water, keep a daily food journal, eat lots of green leafy vegetables, stay away from red meats, prepackaged foods, sugars, sweets (unless sweetened with a healthy substitute) and eat an apple a day.

Drink lots of teas (especially green) and use lots of spices in your foods. And if you like ginger and cinnamon then you may even try both of them in your tea.

"Health Food Cures" is a compilation of over ten years of my personal self-study after a five day hospital stay in 2001 caused by an exhausted immune system from years of stress with no means to relieve the pressure of being a single parent of four children and living on below poverty income in the early nineties.

All Vitamin and Supplement doses are to be taken as the label on the brand of your choice of purchase recommends unless otherwise stated by your doctor. Dosages for specific illnesses of cancer or arthritis are to be taken as suggested in this book unless your doctor tells you otherwise.

I do not recommend coffee enemas though I was advised to have them more then once as a treatment for cancer. I found my deliverance from the hideous disease to be more conservative and user friendly than taking coffee any other way then

orally!

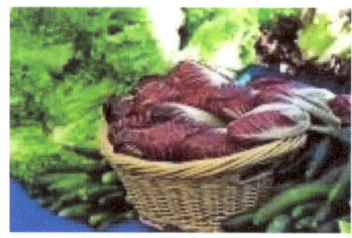

Prone To Arthritis? Counter balance

it with:

Coral Calcium

Vitamin E 400IU

Glucosamine and Chondroitin

Vitamin

Vitamin A 5000 IU

Vitamin D 400 IU

Juniper Berries

Boswellia

Ginger

Turmeric

Black Strap Molasses

MSM Collagen

Alfalfa Hyralonic Acid

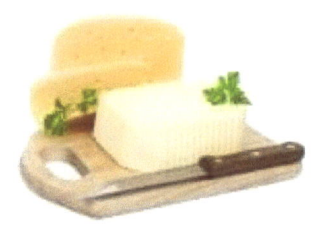

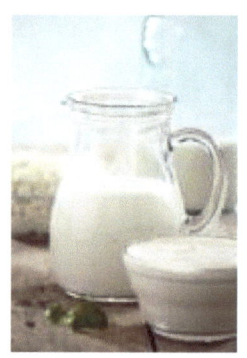

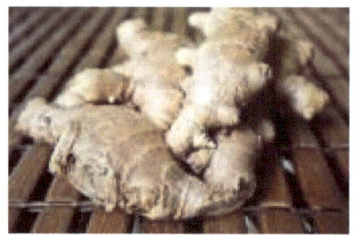

Chemotherapy Treatment Success Enhancers: Ginger greatly decreases nausea in Chemo patients. Selenium before, during and after Chemo greatly increases the success rate of healing as well as greatly decreases the chances of the return of cancer. Gamma Vitamin E fights breast and prostate tumors.

Turmeric shrinks tumors

IP6

Black Strap Molasses turns blood alkaline which greatly reduces the chances of cancer.

Schizandra increase oxygen in blood which also decreases risks of cancer.

1 eight ounce glass of water with ½ teaspoon of baking soda around 3PM each day.

1 eight ounce glass of water with 1 teaspoon of apple cider vinegar each morning upon awaking.

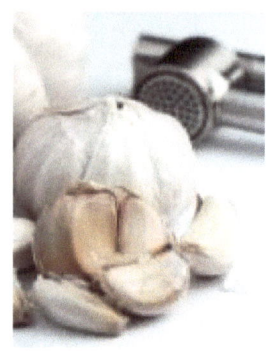

Dissolve Bone Spurs: Acidic

Calcium infused with K2

Chelation Therapy (Remove toxins

build up): Advanced Artery Solution

Saline Colonics

Colloidal Silver

 Angio Prime

 Omega 3

 Lecithin

 Garlic

COQ10

Vitamins D, E, & K,

Pomegranate Juice. (Compliments of

Dr. Hans Petermann)

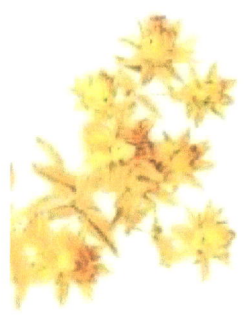

Appetite and Weight Control:

Chromium Picolinate fights certain

types of diabetes.

Tonalin CLA (Safflower Oil is where

some CLA comes from) reduces belly

fat in women

Acai Berry rich in anti-oxidants

Green Tea helps curb appetite, burn

calories and full of cancer fighting

nutrients.

African Mango reduces belly fat.

And Drugs.com says "Research on African mango shows beneficial effects for diabetes and obesity, as well as analgesic, antimicrobial, antioxidant" www.Drugs.com

Alpha Lipoic Acid fights against neuropathy Vinegar helps cleans the body of yeast

Kelp helps fight against virus' when combined with B Complex

Ginsing for added energy and stress relief

Aloe Vera Gel great for constipation and for enzymatic therapy.

Konjac fiber that makes you feel full

Push away from the table a little take

a walk or swim 30 minutes a day.

Hoodia Gardenia greatly suppresses

the appetite.

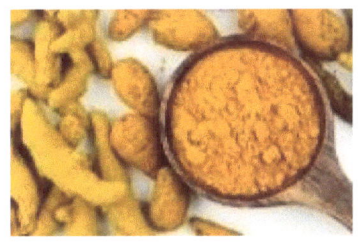

Prostrate or Breast Cancer:

IP6

Gamma Vitamin E 400IU

Selenium

Turmeric

Black Strap Molasses

Schizandra

3 cups of Green tea per day decreases breast cancer by 50%.

2 aspirin per week reduces risk of breast cancer by 20%

Vitamin D decreases risk of breast

cancer by 20%.

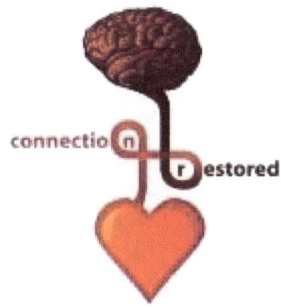

connectio**n** **r** estored

Recently it was reported that Pro football players are at greater risk of early Alzheimer's disease because of the multiple blows to their head. Obese African American women have greater risks and show symptoms of Alzheimer's much earlier than the other study groups.

There are some wonderful natural ways to combat memory loss and stimulate brain health.

Brain Health:

Cumin and black pepper are good to detoxify brain tissue.

You can sprinkle turmeric on your eggs, along with sage, marjoram, basil, and garlic instead of salt.

Alzheimer's:

Ginkgo Biloba

Pregnenolone

Vinpocetine

Coffee

Olive oil & Flax seed Oil

Cod Liver Oil

DHEA

Lecithin

L-Tyrosine

Rhodiola

Ashwagandha

Ginseng

Dl-Phenylalanine

Phosphatidylserine

Cumin

Black Pepper

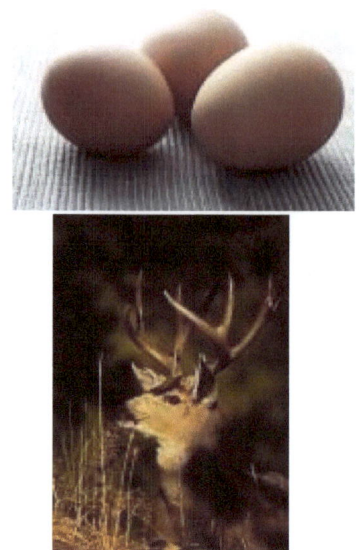

Erectile dysfunction or Impotence:

Ginsing

Deer Antler

Cayenne Pepper

L Arginine

Many drugs that are prescribed for

depression will cause a loss of libido.

Make sure that there is no strife

between you and your spouse. Don't

wander outside of your marriage and

keep your priority on a good

relationship.

Bone Loss:

Coral Calcium

Collagen

Magnesium

Glucosamine and Chondroitin

Boswellia

Vitamin C

Vitamin D 3

Vitamin A

Vitamin E

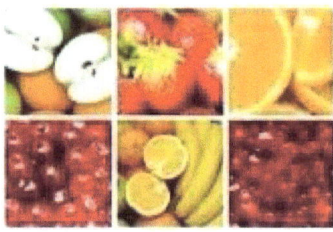

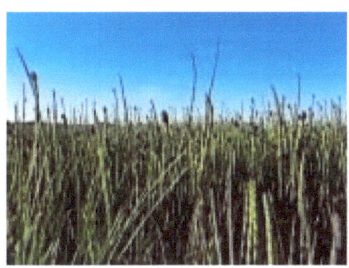

Cartilage Loss

Glucosamine and Chondroitin

 Collagen

Cats Claw

Horse Tail Herb

Vitamin E

Vitamin C

Calcium

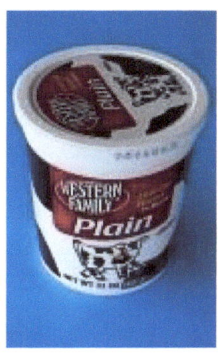

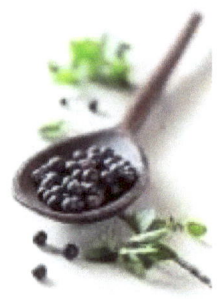

Fibromyalgia:

Juniper Berries

Black Strap Molasses

Ginger is great for digestion and reduces inflammation.

Turmeric shrinks tumors and fights inflammation. Milk thistle detoxifies the liver.

Alfalfa turns blood level back to alkaline to reduce arthritic pain)

Pineapple Bromelain to detoxify and

anti-inflammatory

Tendinitis:

Cats Claw

Alfalfa

Black Strap Molasses (turns blood level back to alkaline reduce arthritic pain)

Ginger

Pineapple or Bromelain (will detoxify and act as an all-natural anti-inflammatory)

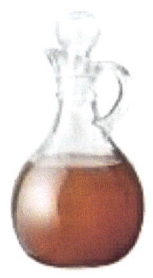

Chronic Fatigue:

B-Complex and Kelp

Plain Yogurt

Apple Cider Vinegar

Acidophiles (detoxify and anti-

inflammatory)

Pro Biotics

Phosphatidylserine stops release of

cortisol and helps with depression.

Rest! A Stress free environment until

complete health and wellbeing are

restored for as long as necessary
(depends on how chronic} It could
take up to ten years in extreme cases
where the immune system has shut
down. Medical Science has proven
that stress causes cancer. They have
been teaching that in Modern
Psychology since the early nineties.
And they are still teaching it today in
Social Science and Social Behavior
Classes as I was a student of
Psychology Holmes Community
College Ridgeland, MS. In the early
nineties and once again in 2011 I took
another class on May 16, 2011 -

"Stressed to the Nines: The Hard

Truth about Anxiety and You "

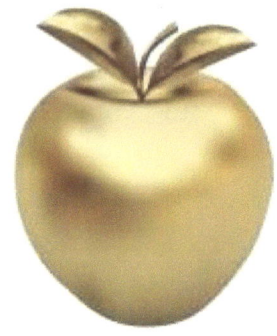

Constipation:

Cascara Sagrada

Senna

Wormwood parasite cleanser

Black Walnut Hull parasite cleanser

Slippery Elm

Konjac fiber that makes you feel full

Old World Botanicals is a great place

to find most everything mentioned in

this book.

Esophagitis, Indigestion or Heart Burn:

Orange peel stops acid indigestion much faster and better than prescription ulcer medicine without the harmful side effects.

Licorice use like a sweetener in tea as a sugar substitute.

Bromelain

Aloc Vcra gcl

Apple Pectin or the skin of an apple.

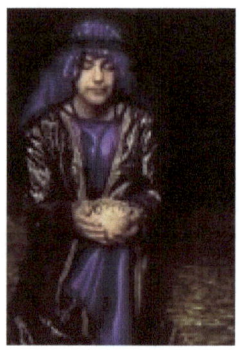

Pain Management & Anti

Inflammatory: Ginger

Turmeric

Boswellia

Black Strap Molasses

Fish Oil

Bromelain

Alfalfa

Yeast Detoxification:

Plain Yogurt on empty stomach

Apple Cider Vinegar

Pau D' Arco

Pro Biotics Oregano oil

Caprylic Acid

Beta Glucan

Here is another great place to get

answers for [Curing Yeast](http://kimig.tripod.com/yeastcures/)

http://kimig.tripod.com/yeastcures/

Parasite Cleansing:

Crushed Papaya seeds

Black Walnut Hull

Cilantro

Garlic

Worm wood

Earl Grey

Bergamot tea

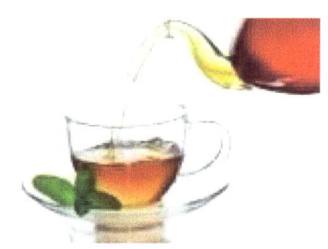

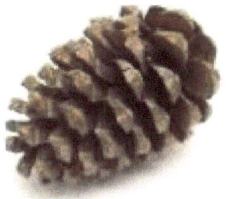

Hair loss:

Collagen

Horse Tail

B-Complex

Vitamin E

Pine Bark

Exfoliate scalp with honey, sugar and conditioner; apply in circular motion let sit for fifteen minutes then wash as normal.

Immune Deficiency:

Vitamin C

Selenium

Zinc

Colloidal Silver

Copper

Vitamin B Complex

Kelp

Vitamin E

Beta Glucan

DMG Mushrooms:

Maitake, Shiitake, Reishi,

Human Growth Hormone

Blue Berries

Grapeseed Extract

Manganese

Acai Berry

Dark Chocolate

Coffee

Co Q 10

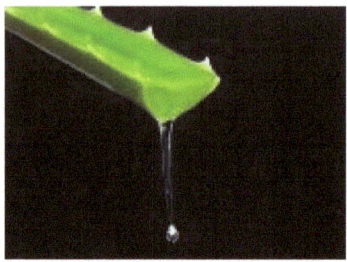

Type 2 Diabetes control:

Hoodia Gardenia

African Mango

Chromium picolinate

Pine Nut

Tonalin CLA

Acai Berry

Green Tea

Alpha Lipoic Acid

Apple Cider Vinegar

Kelp B Complex

Ginsing

Aloe Vera Gel

Konjac (fiber that makes you feel full)

Push away from the table a little take

a walk or swim 30 minutes a day

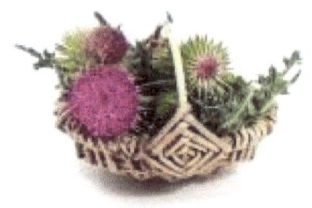

Hepatitis or other liver disease:

Milk Thistle

Burdock Root

Hyssop Red Clover

Green Vegetables

Echinacea

Insomnia:

Collagen

Dong Qui

Valerian Root

Magnesium

Melatonin (naturally found in Milk,

Turkey, or Chicken)

Wrinkle Reduction:

Natural Alpha Hydroxy ie apple juice,

sugar, or honey & brown sugar

applied to the wrinkles at bedtime.

Remove with Corn meal facial scrub

in the morning. Use plain coconut oil

to moisturize.

Dark Circle Removal :

1 drop of Sweet Orange combined

with 5 drops of grape seed oil.

To reduce swelling around the eyes:

Use 1/2 teaspoon of Preparation H

cream only (not the oily ointment)

and be sure not to get it near or in the

eye. Apply to effected area.

To help heal the blood vessels around

the eye use 2 Arnica tablets dissolved

in 1 tablespoon of water apply one

drop under effected eye.

Anxiety:

Lavender tea

Skullcap tea

Valerian Root

Dong Qui (take when needed or

during ministration)

Phosphatidylserine (stops the release

of cortisol)

Blood Clots, Restless Leg Syndrome

or Varicose Veins:

Horse Chestnut

Aspirin

Vinegar rub downs

Ginger

Garlic

Onions

Niacin

Fever Few

Schizandra

Shepherds purse

Butchers broom

Lumbrokinase (Chinese Earthworm enzyme that eats blood clots it is also great for allergies)

Poor Circulation:

Horse Chestnut

Schizandra

Aspirin

Hawthorne Berry

Fever Few

Niacin

Cardiovascular body movements.
Recently medical statistics revealed
that people with poor circulation are
at higher risk for heart disease and
stroke. It is very serious and most
heart tests do not reveal any problems
in people with poor circulation when
they are experiencing chest pain.

Be sure and see a medical doctor if you have chest pain. Butchers broom and Horse chestnut combined with Hawthorne Berry and Aspirin are more than enough to take the pain and inflammation away.

However, Hawthorne Berry is a very potent blood thinner and you must ask your doctor before taking it. You cannot take Hawthorn Berry prior to having any surgical procedures.

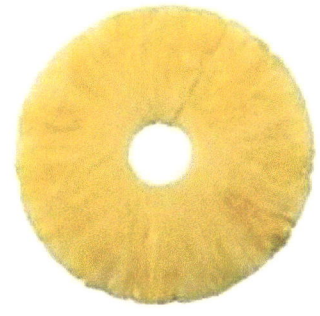

Inflammation:

Ginger

Turmeric

Boswellia

Black Strap Molasses

Willow Bark or better known as

Aspirin Bromelain or better known as

Pineapple

Fish Oil (Recent studies have linked

inflammation to heart disease and

cancer)

Sinusitis:

Xylitol nasal wash

Mullein

Olive leaf

Saline nasal wash (1 Quart of (distilled) water only, 2 tablespoons of canning salt 1 tablespoon of baking soda warmed to room temperature)

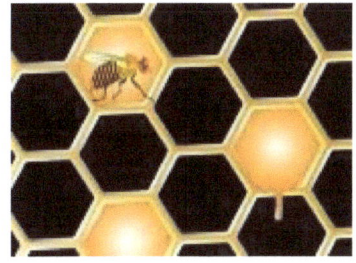

Allergies:

Bromelain

Mug wort

Bee Propolis

Mullein

Lumbrokinase (Chinese Earthworm

enzyme that eats blood clots)

Cholesterol Control:

Garlic

Ex. Virgin Olive oil

Niacin

Polycosanol

Remove all butter and vegetable oil from your food. Replace butter with Extra Virgin Olive oil for a spread on your toast or potatoes. And you can also use the olive oil in your salad dressings. Switch to Coconut oil to cook all your food with. This will eliminate bad cholesterol and help build up good cholesterol.

Heart Health:

CO Q10

Niacin

Garlic Fish Oil

Hawthorn Berry

Ribose

Horse Chestnut

Magnesium

Calcium

Ecotrin coated Aspirin

Polycosanol

Lumbrokinase (Chinese Earthworm

enzyme that eats arterial blood clots)

Recently medical statistics revealed

that people with poor circulation are

at higher risk for heart disease and

stroke. It is very serious and most

heart tests do not reveal any problems

in people with poor circulation when

they are experiencing chest pain.

Be sure and see a medical doctor if

you have chest pain. Butchers broom

and Horse chestnut combined with

Hawthorne Berry and Aspirin are

more than enough to get rid of pain.

Anti-Clotting:

Ginger

Garlic

Onions

Shepherds purse or soldiers tea.

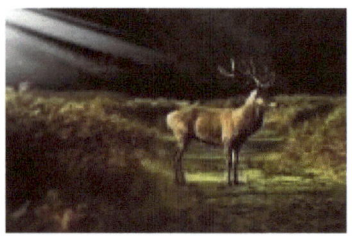

Deer velvet antler Has been scientifically proven to provide the following benefits:

Combating Cancer

Improving the Immune System functions Improving Athletic Performance

Stamina and Strength

Improving Muscle Recovery from muscle stress after exercise.

Also an excellent natural supplement for Women's Health.

Providing Vitality and Anti-aging properties for Seniors.

Can be used as an alternative natural supplement for Bodybuilding and Weight Training.

Has an excellent source of Growth Factors including IGF-1 & IGF-2.

Improves and enhances sexual functioning for both men and women.

It's a natural supplement for Arthritis.

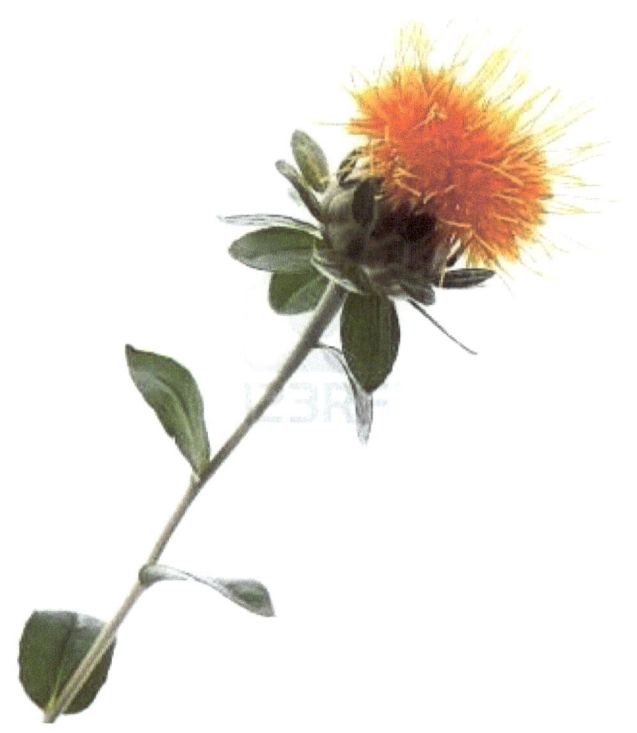

Relieve Depression:

Phosphatidylserine

5 HTP

St. John's Wart

Dill

Majoram

Saffron

Nutmeg

Peppermint

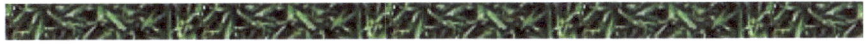

Everyone benefits in health and in

weight control when they switch ALL

butters, vegetable oils, or fat back

grease and replace all of those with

Olive oil on toast, popcorn, salads,

and switch to coconut oil for cooking.

You must not cook olive oil at high

temperatures because it causes

chemical structure to mutate and

instead of being healthy it becomes a

health hazard. On the other hand,

Coconut oil can be cooked at high

temperatures and it is very healthy just as olive oils are.

You will also find that there are many sugar substitutes such as honey or Xylitol that is much better for your immune system and the Xylitol will help fight cavities while trimming your waist. It looks and feels exactly like sugar does.

Recently Medical Research has discovered that Chronic Inflammation greatly increased the risk for women in stroke and heart attacks or heart disease. There is a new simple test to determine how much inflammation is in your blood.

See your physician to see if that is something that you need at this time. There are simple anti-inflammatory herbs and remedies mentioned above. You can also start your day out with pineapple for breakfast. The enzymes in the pineapple help to breakdown the protein cells in the walls of cancer formation.

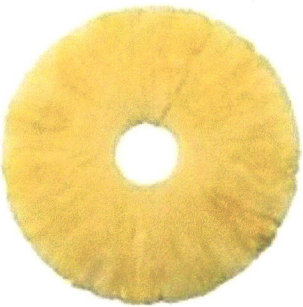

These are just a few simple ways that we have seen to bring great improvement for health naturally after years of research.

We use homeopathic remedies, herbs, teas, and supplements. We believe that the best cure is from the Great physician and creator the Great God Jehovah.

And that He has given herbs and nutrients that help us to maintain health by obeying His word and taking care of our temples (bodies) by respecting them with good health care practices.

One thing we all need each and every day of our lives is health!

Many are over stressed in over drive and have taxed the immune system to the point that it is shutting down.

In some cases their bodies have excreted so much adrenaline from the Adrenalin Gland till there is not anymore "fight or flight" Epinephrine [Epinephrine - Epinephrine (also referred to as adrenaline;) is a hormone and neurotransmitter.

It is a catecholamine, a sympathomimetic monoamine extracted from the amino acids: phenylalanine and tyrosine.

(Referring to the adrenal gland, which sits atop the kidneys and secretes epinephrine) When this happens our body becomes vulnerable to disease. This will keep causing the body to continual release cortisol. It will wear down the immune system. Cortisol is what causes women to have too much stored fat in the belly. And maybe related to the rise in heart disease in women.

In some cases, it is nearly impossible to stop this downward spiral of destruction because the chemical has such a profound effect on our brains that in turn effects our entire lives. But even the worst case scenario can

find hope in providing the body what
it has to have to function properly.

Let us help you to regain control of
your health! Using all natural and
botanical herbs combined with
common sense, daily supplements of
vitamins, minerals, and a healthy diet
are basics that get the body back on
track to optimal health.

Rest is essential for the healing
properties to manifest speedily. And
a healthy environment is also
important to get optimal results. We
use a Healing Approach to master
Disease Control and operate in

Preventive Health care as well as

Traditional and

Conventional Medicine applied

conservatively.

The Bible tells us that we are to obey

our physicians and we would never

counsel against your own doctors'

advice. Most of our remedies can be

found the kitchen cabinets anywhere,

U.S.A.

And if there is a concern about a

specific herb we would ask that you

consult with your physician.

Our goal is to help you feel better,

look better, and live longer! We only

provide Natural and Homeopathic Remedies. And for the most part, our goal of optimal health is obtained best by Preventive Health Care.

Natural Remedies are generally less expensive than prescription drugs, less side effects, and usually have more benefits than just healing a specific disease. For instance the treatment for fighting cancer also fights inflammation.

These herbs in and of itself is not the cure. But combined with a healthy lifestyle pleasing to God and eating properly, that healing will be activated. There are some foods that have to be abstained from and other

foods that need to be partook of.

It is like if you were eating foods

with high calories and no vitamin or

nutritional value, we need you to now

do just the opposite, high vitamin and

nutritional value with very few

calories. Spices and Teas are very

beneficial in the healing process. In

the Consultation we can determine

which ones are best for you.

www.ingramcontent.com/pod-product-compliance
Lightning Source LLC
Chambersburg PA
CBHW050809290526
45792CB00001B/50